This Jo

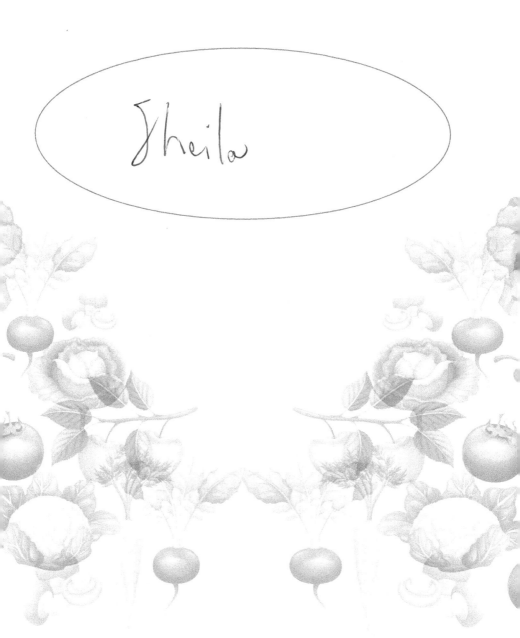

Sheila

Use this daily journal and log book to accompany your journey on the new System 20 health plan found online at https://www.doctoroz.com/feature/system-20

Disclosure:
I am not affiliated with the website or the program.

About Intermittent Fasting

Intermittent fasting can be traced back to the days of the caveman due to food scarcity, but according to research this ancient survival adaption can be an effective tool for weight loss, blood sugar and blood pressure control, and improving heart health. [1]

When we're in the fasted state (12 hours after your last meal) our insulin levels go down, and our fat cells can then release their stored sugar, to be used as energy. Thus, we burn fat.

If you get in a long enough fast overnight, you can burn through all your body's carb storage (called glycogen) and start burning fat. [2]

FAVORITE TIPS

- Visit the website: **lift.foundation** for a free guided meditation you can do daily.

- Download the **Sleepscore app** by Sleepscore labs to monitor sleep patterns.

- Make a big pot of soup to eat in a pinch - for creamy soups use canned coconut milk instead of heavy cream.

- Drink plenty of water.

- Skip nightime snacks & alcohol.

- Power off the electronics 1 hr before sleep.

- Keep a daily gratitude log.

Sources:
1. https://thedo.osteopathic.org/2019/01/intermittent-fasting-can-we-fast-our-way-to-better-health/
2. https://www.doctoroz.com/gallery/15-day-plan-reset-your-body?gallery=true&page=2

Notes

Breakfast @ 11:00 AM
eat till 7:00 PM

before 11:00 AM {
do meditation

cardio

tea with MCT oil
}

no caffine after 3:00 PM

Here's an example of what a 16:8 fast looks like.

You can adjust the 8 hour eating window according to your schedule.

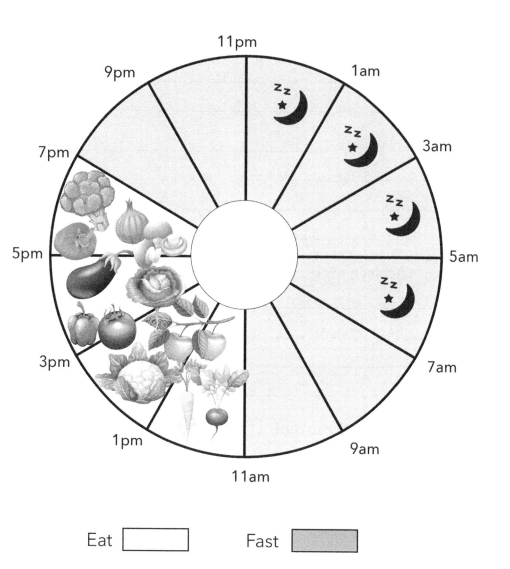

Eat ☐   Fast ▨

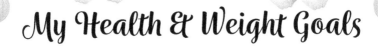

My Health & Weight Goals

My short term goals: _____

_____

_____

_____

My long term goals: _____

_____

_____

_____

How will I achieve my goals: *(for example: fast, eliminate certain foods, exercise)*

_____

_____

_____

_____

Why is this important to me? _____

_____

_____

_____

_____

_____

_____

Starting Measurements

Date _____

Neck _____ "

Arm _____ "

Chest _____ "

Hips _____ "

Belly _____ "

Thigh _____ "

Weight _____

BP _____

REPEAT AFTER ME:

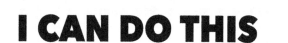

I CAN DO THIS

CHEAT DAY? Y N	# DAILY TRACKING SHEET	WEIGHT

Today I begin again: _____
DATE

🌙 🌙 🌙 🌙 🌙 LAST NIGHT 🌙 🌙 🌙 🌙 🌙

My wakeup goal time was: _____

My actual wakeup time was: _____

Total hours I slept was: _____

SLEEP SCORE

○ I had a very deep sleep

○ I tossed and turned for hours

TODAY

DRANK Coffee or Tea w/MCT Oil: ○ YES ○ NO

MEDITATED: ○ YES ○ NO | EXERCISED: ○ YES ○ NO

WHAT I CONSUMED DURING MY 8 HOUR EATING WINDOW:

○ 1 TBSP Braggs Apple Cider Vinegar before brunch

___am BRUNCH Greens _____ Beans _____ Protein _____

___pm AFTERNOON SNACK _____

○ 1 TBSP Braggs Apple Cider Vinegar before dinner

___pm DINNER Greens _____ Beans _____ Protein _____

___pm EVENING SNACK or BERRIES _____

Alchoholic Beverages? ○ Yes ○ No _____

WATER ☐ ☐ ☐ ☐ ☐ ☐ ☐ ☐

CROSS OFF A GLASS EVERY TIME YOU DRINK 8OZ OF WATER

WHAT I CONSUMED *AFTER* MY 8 HOUR EATING WINDOW:

○ I had a phone conversation today with: _____

○ I turned off electronics one hour before bed time at: _____

Today I am especially thankful for: _____

CHEAT DAY?	# DAILY TRACKING SHEET	WEIGHT
Y N	Today I begin again: _____ DATE	

☾ ☾ ☾ ☾ ☾ **LAST NIGHT** ☾ ☾ ☾ ☾ ☾

My wakeup goal time was: _____

My actual wakeup time was: _____

Total hours I slept was: _____

SLEEP SCORE

○ I had a very deep sleep

○ I tossed and turned for hours

TODAY

DRANK Coffee or Tea w/MCT Oil: ○ YES   ○ NO

MEDITATED: ○ YES LiFT foundation ○ NO | EXERCISED: ○ YES ○ NO

WHAT I CONSUMED DURING MY 8 HOUR EATING WINDOW:

○ 1 TBSP Braggs Apple Cider Vinegar before brunch

___am BRUNCH   Greens _____   Beans _____   Protein _____

___pm AFTERNOON SNACK _____

○ 1 TBSP Braggs Apple Cider Vinegar before dinner

___pm DINNER Greens _____   Beans _____   Protein _____

___pm EVENING SNACK or BERRIES _____

Alchoholic Beverages? ○ Yes ○ No _____

WATER ▯ ▯ ▯ ▯ ▯ ▯ ▯ ▯

CROSS OFF A GLASS EVERY TIME YOU DRINK 8OZ OF WATER

WHAT I CONSUMED *AFTER* MY 8 HOUR EATING WINDOW:

○ I had a phone conversation today with: _____

○ I turned off electronics one hour before bed time at: _____

Today I am especially thankful for: _____

CHEAT DAY?	# DAILY TRACKING SHEET	WEIGHT
Y N	Today I begin again: _____ DATE	

🌙🌙🌙🌙🌙 LAST NIGHT 🌙🌙🌙🌙🌙

My wakeup goal time was: _____

My actual wakeup time was: _____

Total hours I slept was: _____

SLEEP SCORE

○ I had a very deep sleep

○ I tossed and turned for hours

TODAY

DRANK Coffee or Tea w/MCT Oil: ○ YES   ○ NO

MEDITATED: ○ YES *LIFT* foundation ○ NO   EXERCISED: ○ YES   ○ NO

WHAT I CONSUMED DURING MY 8 HOUR EATING WINDOW:

○ 1 TBSP Braggs Apple Cider Vinegar before brunch

___am BRUNCH   Greens _____   Beans _____   Protein _____

___pm AFTERNOON SNACK _____

○ 1 TBSP Braggs Apple Cider Vinegar before dinner

___pm DINNER Greens _____   Beans _____   Protein _____

___pm EVENING SNACK or BERRIES _____

Alchoholic Beverages? ○ Yes ○ No _____

WATER ⬜ ⬜ ⬜ ⬜ ⬜ ⬜ ⬜ ⬜

CROSS OFF A GLASS EVERY TIME YOU DRINK 8OZ OF WATER

WHAT I CONSUMED *AFTER* MY 8 HOUR EATING WINDOW:

○ I had a phone conversation today with: _____

○ I turned off electronics one hour before bed time at: _____

Today I am especially thankful for: _____

CHEAT DAY?	# DAILY TRACKING SHEET	WEIGHT
Y N		

Today I begin again: _____
                                          DATE

🌙🌙🌙🌙🌙 LAST NIGHT 🌙🌙🌙🌙🌙

My wakeup goal time was: _____

My actual wakeup time was: _____

Total hours I slept was: _____

SLEEP SCORE

○ I had a very deep sleep
○ I tossed and turned for hours

TODAY

DRANK Coffee or Tea w/MCT Oil: ○ YES   ○ NO

MEDITATED: ○ YES 🦁LIFT foundation ○ NO | EXERCISED: ○ YES ○ NO

WHAT I CONSUMED DURING MY 8 HOUR EATING WINDOW:

○ 1 TBSP Braggs Apple Cider Vinegar before brunch

___am BRUNCH   Greens _____   Beans _____   Protein _____

___pm AFTERNOON SNACK _____

○ 1 TBSP Braggs Apple Cider Vinegar before dinner

___pm DINNER Greens _____   Beans _____   Protein _____

___pm EVENING SNACK or BERRIES _____

Alchoholic Beverages? ○ Yes ○ No _____

WATER   ⊔ ⊔ ⊔ ⊔ ⊔ ⊔ ⊔ ⊔

CROSS OFF A GLASS EVERY TIME YOU DRINK 8OZ OF WATER

WHAT I CONSUMED *AFTER* MY 8 HOUR EATING WINDOW:

○ I had a phone conversation today with: _____

○ I turned off electronics one hour before bed time at: _____

Today I am especially thankful for: _____

∽ 11 ∽

DAILY TRACKING SHEET

WEIGHT

Today I begin again: _____
DATE

LAST NIGHT

My wakeup goal time was: _____

My actual wakeup time was: _____

Total hours I slept was: _____

SLEEP SCORE

○ I had a very deep sleep

○ I tossed and turned for hours

TODAY

DRANK Coffee or Tea w/MCT Oil: ○ YES   ○ NO

MEDITATED: ○ YES 🐾LIFT foundation ○ NO | EXERCISED: ○ YES ○ NO

WHAT I CONSUMED DURING MY 8 HOUR EATING WINDOW:

○ 1 TBSP Braggs Apple Cider Vinegar before brunch

___am BRUNCH   Greens _____   Beans _____   Protein _____

___pm AFTERNOON SNACK _____

○ 1 TBSP Braggs Apple Cider Vinegar before dinner

___pm DINNER Greens _____   Beans _____   Protein _____

___pm EVENING SNACK or BERRIES _____

Alchoholic Beverages? ○ Yes ○ No _____

WATER ☐ ☐ ☐ ☐ ☐ ☐ ☐ ☐

CROSS OFF A GLASS EVERY TIME YOU DRINK 8OZ OF WATER

WHAT I CONSUMED *AFTER* MY 8 HOUR EATING WINDOW:

○ I had a phone conversation today with: _____

○ I turned off electronics one hour before bed time at: _____

Today I am especially thankful for: _____

∽ 12 ∽

DAILY TRACKING SHEET

Today I begin again: _____
DATE

🌙 🌙 🌙 🌙 🌙 LAST NIGHT 🌙 🌙 🌙 🌙 🌙

My wakeup goal time was: _____

My actual wakeup time was: _____

Total hours I slept was: _____

SLEEP SCORE

○ I had a very deep sleep
○ I tossed and turned for hours

TODAY

DRANK Coffee or Tea w/MCT Oil: ○ YES   ○ NO

MEDITATED: ○ YES LiFT foundation ○ NO | EXERCISED: ○ YES ○ NO

WHAT I CONSUMED DURING MY 8 HOUR EATING WINDOW:

○ 1 TBSP Braggs Apple Cider Vinegar before brunch

___am BRUNCH   Greens _____ Beans _____ Protein _____

___pm AFTERNOON SNACK _____

○ 1 TBSP Braggs Apple Cider Vinegar before dinner

___pm DINNER Greens _____ Beans _____ Protein _____

___pm EVENING SNACK or BERRIES _____

Alchoholic Beverages? ○ Yes ○ No _____

WATER ▯ ▯ ▯ ▯ ▯ ▯ ▯ ▯

CROSS OFF A GLASS EVERY TIME YOU DRINK 8OZ OF WATER

WHAT I CONSUMED *AFTER* MY 8 HOUR EATING WINDOW:

○ I had a phone conversation today with: _____

○ I turned off electronics one hour before bed time at: _____

Today I am especially thankful for: _____

∽ 13 ∽

DAILY TRACKING SHEET

WEIGHT

Today I begin again: _____
DATE

🌙 🌙 🌙 🌙 🌙 LAST NIGHT 🌙 🌙 🌙 🌙 🌙

My wakeup goal time was: _____

My actual wakeup time was: _____

Total hours I slept was: _____

| SLEEP SCORE | ○ I had a very deep sleep
○ I tossed and turned for hours |

TODAY

DRANK Coffee or Tea w/MCT Oil: ○ YES   ○ NO

MEDITATED: ○ YES *LiFT foundation* ○ NO | EXERCISED: ○ YES ○ NO

WHAT I CONSUMED DURING MY 8 HOUR EATING WINDOW:

○ 1 TBSP Braggs Apple Cider Vinegar before brunch

___am BRUNCH   Greens _____   Beans _____   Protein _____

___pm AFTERNOON SNACK _____

○ 1 TBSP Braggs Apple Cider Vinegar before dinner

___pm DINNER Greens _____   Beans _____   Protein _____

___pm EVENING SNACK or BERRIES _____

Alchoholic Beverages? ○ Yes ○ No _____

WATER ▯ ▯ ▯ ▯ ▯ ▯ ▯ ▯

CROSS OFF A GLASS EVERY TIME YOU DRINK 8OZ OF WATER

WHAT I CONSUMED *AFTER* MY 8 HOUR EATING WINDOW:

_____

○ I had a phone conversation today with: _____

○ I turned off electronics one hour before bed time at: _____

Today I am especially thankful for: _____

Measurements (After 1 week)

Date _____

Neck _____ "

Arm _____ "

Chest _____ "

Belly _____ "

Hips _____ "

Thigh _____ "

Weight _____

BP _____

When you feel like

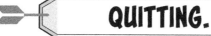

QUITTING.

Think about

WHY

you started.

Notes & Reflections

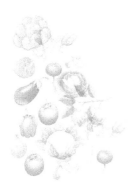

DAILY TRACKING SHEET

WEIGHT

Today I begin again: _____
DATE

🌙 🌙 🌙 🌙 🌙 LAST NIGHT 🌙 🌙 🌙 🌙 🌙

My wakeup goal time was: _____

My actual wakeup time was: _____

Total hours I slept was: _____

SLEEP SCORE

○ I had a very deep sleep

○ I tossed and turned for hours

TODAY

DRANK Coffee or Tea w/MCT Oil: ○ YES   ○ NO

MEDITATED: ○ YES LiFT Foundation ○ NO | EXERCISED: ○ YES ○ NO

WHAT I CONSUMED DURING MY 8 HOUR EATING WINDOW:

○ 1 TBSP Braggs Apple Cider Vinegar before brunch

___am BRUNCH   Greens _____   Beans _____   Protein _____

___pm AFTERNOON SNACK _____

○ 1 TBSP Braggs Apple Cider Vinegar before dinner

___pm DINNER Greens _____   Beans _____   Protein _____

___pm EVENING SNACK or BERRIES _____

Alchoholic Beverages? ○ Yes   ○ No _____

WATER ⬜ ⬜ ⬜ ⬜ ⬜ ⬜ ⬜ ⬜

CROSS OFF A GLASS EVERY TIME YOU DRINK 8OZ OF WATER

WHAT I CONSUMED AFTER MY 8 HOUR EATING WINDOW:

○ I had a phone conversation today with: _____

○ I turned off electronics one hour before bed time at: _____

Today I am especially thankful for: _____

DAILY TRACKING SHEET

WEIGHT

Today I begin again: _____
DATE

🌙🌙🌙🌙🌙 LAST NIGHT 🌙🌙🌙🌙🌙

My wakeup goal time was: _____

My actual wakeup time was: _____

Total hours I slept was: _____

SLEEP SCORE

○ I had a very deep sleep
○ I tossed and turned for hours

TODAY

DRANK Coffee or Tea w/MCT Oil: ○ YES   ○ NO

MEDITATED: ○ YES LiFT foundation ○ NO   EXERCISED: ○ YES ○ NO

WHAT I CONSUMED DURING MY 8 HOUR EATING WINDOW:

○ 1 TBSP Braggs Apple Cider Vinegar before brunch

___am BRUNCH   Greens _____   Beans _____   Protein _____

___pm AFTERNOON SNACK _____

○ 1 TBSP Braggs Apple Cider Vinegar before dinner

___pm DINNER Greens _____   Beans _____   Protein _____

___pm EVENING SNACK or BERRIES _____

Alchoholic Beverages? ○ Yes ○ No _____

WATER [ ] [ ] [ ] [ ] [ ] [ ] [ ] [ ]

CROSS OFF A GLASS EVERY TIME YOU DRINK 8OZ OF WATER

WHAT I CONSUMED *AFTER* MY 8 HOUR EATING WINDOW:

○ I had a phone conversation today with: _____

○ I turned off electronics one hour before bed time at: _____

Today I am especially thankful for: _____

DAILY TRACKING SHEET

Today I begin again: _____
DATE

🌙🌙🌙🌙🌙 LAST NIGHT 🌙🌙🌙🌙🌙

My wakeup goal time was: _____

My actual wakeup time was: _____

Total hours I slept was: _____

SLEEP SCORE

○ I had a very deep sleep

○ I tossed and turned for hours

TODAY

DRANK Coffee or Tea w/MCT Oil: ○ YES   ○ NO

MEDITATED: ○ YES *LIFT* foundation ○ NO | EXERCISED: ○ YES ○ NO

WHAT I CONSUMED DURING MY 8 HOUR EATING WINDOW:

○ 1 TBSP Braggs Apple Cider Vinegar before brunch

___am BRUNCH   Greens _____   Beans _____   Protein _____

___pm AFTERNOON SNACK _____

○ 1 TBSP Braggs Apple Cider Vinegar before dinner

___pm DINNER Greens _____   Beans _____   Protein _____

___pm EVENING SNACK or BERRIES _____

Alchoholic Beverages? ○ Yes ○ No _____

WATER ☐ ☐ ☐ ☐ ☐ ☐ ☐ ☐

CROSS OFF A GLASS EVERY TIME YOU DRINK 8OZ OF WATER

WHAT I CONSUMED *AFTER* MY 8 HOUR EATING WINDOW:

○ I had a phone conversation today with: _____

○ I turned off electronics one hour before bed time at: _____

Today I am especially thankful for: _____

DAILY TRACKING SHEET

Today I begin again: _____
DATE

🌙 🌙 🌙 🌙 🌙 LAST NIGHT 🌙 🌙 🌙 🌙 🌙

My wakeup goal time was: _____

My actual wakeup time was: _____

Total hours I slept was: _____

SLEEP SCORE

○ I had a very deep sleep

○ I tossed and turned for hours

TODAY

DRANK Coffee or Tea w/MCT Oil: ○ YES ○ NO

MEDITATED: ○ YES LiFT foundation ○ NO | EXERCISED: ○ YES ○ NO

WHAT I CONSUMED DURING MY 8 HOUR EATING WINDOW:

○ 1 TBSP Braggs Apple Cider Vinegar before brunch

___am BRUNCH   Greens _____   Beans _____   Protein _____

___pm AFTERNOON SNACK _____

○ 1 TBSP Braggs Apple Cider Vinegar before dinner

___pm DINNER Greens _____   Beans _____   Protein _____

___pm EVENING SNACK or BERRIES _____

Alchoholic Beverages? ○ Yes ○ No _____

WATER [ ] [ ] [ ] [ ] [ ] [ ] [ ]

CROSS OFF A GLASS EVERY TIME YOU DRINK 8OZ OF WATER

WHAT I CONSUMED *AFTER* MY 8 HOUR EATING WINDOW:

_____

○ I had a phone conversation today with: _____

○ I turned off electronics one hour before bed time at: _____

Today I am especially thankful for: _____

DAILY TRACKING SHEET

Today I begin again: _____
                        DATE

🌙 🌙 🌙 🌙 🌙 LAST NIGHT 🌙 🌙 🌙 🌙 🌙

My wakeup goal time was: _____

My actual wakeup time was: _____

Total hours I slept was: _____

SLEEP SCORE

○ I had a very deep sleep

○ I tossed and turned for hours

TODAY

DRANK Coffee or Tea w/MCT Oil: ○ YES   ○ NO

MEDITATED: ○ YES **LiFT** foundation ○ NO | EXERCISED: ○ YES ○ NO

WHAT I CONSUMED DURING MY 8 HOUR EATING WINDOW:

○ 1 TBSP Braggs Apple Cider Vinegar before brunch

___am BRUNCH   Greens _____   Beans _____   Protein _____

___pm AFTERNOON SNACK _____

○ 1 TBSP Braggs Apple Cider Vinegar before dinner

___pm DINNER Greens _____   Beans _____   Protein _____

___pm EVENING SNACK or BERRIES _____

Alchoholic Beverages? ○ Yes ○ No _____

WATER ☐ ☐ ☐ ☐ ☐ ☐ ☐ ☐

CROSS OFF A GLASS EVERY TIME YOU DRINK 8OZ OF WATER

WHAT I CONSUMED *AFTER* MY 8 HOUR EATING WINDOW:

○ I had a phone conversation today with: _____

○ I turned off electronics one hour before bed time at: _____

Today I am especially thankful for: _____

DAILY TRACKING SHEET

CHEAT DAY?		WEIGHT
Y N		

Today I begin again: _____
DATE

🌙🌙🌙🌙🌙 LAST NIGHT 🌙🌙🌙🌙🌙

My wakeup goal time was: _____

My actual wakeup time was: _____

Total hours I slept was: _____

SLEEP SCORE

○ I had a very deep sleep

○ I tossed and turned for hours

TODAY

DRANK Coffee or Tea w/MCT Oil: ○ YES   ○ NO

MEDITATED: ○ YES 🐾LIFT foundation ○ NO   EXERCISED: ○ YES ○ NO

WHAT I CONSUMED DURING MY 8 HOUR EATING WINDOW:

○ 1 TBSP Braggs Apple Cider Vinegar before brunch

___am BRUNCH   Greens _____   Beans _____   Protein _____

___pm AFTERNOON SNACK _____

○ 1 TBSP Braggs Apple Cider Vinegar before dinner

___pm DINNER Greens _____   Beans _____   Protein _____

___pm EVENING SNACK or BERRIES _____

Alchoholic Beverages? ○ Yes ○ No _____

WATER ☐ ☐ ☐ ☐ ☐ ☐ ☐ ☐
CROSS OFF A GLASS EVERY TIME YOU DRINK 8OZ OF WATER

WHAT I CONSUMED *AFTER* MY 8 HOUR EATING WINDOW:

_____

○ I had a phone conversation today with: _____

○ I turned off electronics one hour before bed time at: _____

Today I am especially thankful for: _____

DAILY TRACKING SHEET

WEIGHT

Today I begin again: _____
DATE

🌙 🌙 🌙 🌙 🌙 LAST NIGHT 🌙 🌙 🌙 🌙 🌙

My wakeup goal time was: _____

My actual wakeup time was: _____

Total hours I slept was: _____

SLEEP SCORE

○ I had a very deep sleep
○ I tossed and turned for hours

TODAY

DRANK Coffee or Tea w/MCT Oil: ○ YES ○ NO

MEDITATED: ○ YES LiFT foundation ○ NO | EXERCISED: ○ YES ○ NO

WHAT I CONSUMED DURING MY 8 HOUR EATING WINDOW:

○ 1 TBSP Braggs Apple Cider Vinegar before brunch

___am BRUNCH   Greens _____   Beans _____   Protein _____

___pm AFTERNOON SNACK _____

○ 1 TBSP Braggs Apple Cider Vinegar before dinner

___pm DINNER Greens _____   Beans _____   Protein _____

___pm EVENING SNACK or BERRIES _____

Alchoholic Beverages? ○ Yes ○ No _____

WATER ▢ ▢ ▢ ▢ ▢ ▢ ▢ ▢

CROSS OFF A GLASS EVERY TIME YOU DRINK 8OZ OF WATER

WHAT I CONSUMED *AFTER* MY 8 HOUR EATING WINDOW:

○ I had a phone conversation today with: _____

○ I turned off electronics one hour before bed time at: _____

Today I am especially thankful for: _____

Measurements (After 2 weeks)

Date _____

Neck _____ "

Arm _____ "

Hips _____ "

Chest _____ "

Belly _____ "

Thigh _____ "

Weight _____

BP _____

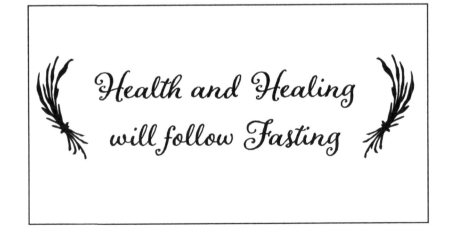

Health and Healing will follow Fasting

Notes & Reflections

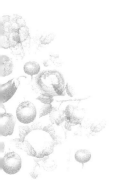
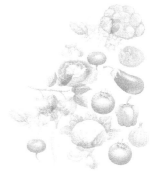

DAILY TRACKING SHEET

Today I begin again: _____
DATE

☾ ☾ ☾ ☾ ☾ LAST NIGHT ☾ ☾ ☾ ☾ ☾

My wakeup goal time was: _____

My actual wakeup time was: _____

Total hours I slept was: _____

SLEEP SCORE

○ I had a very deep sleep

○ I tossed and turned for hours

TODAY

DRANK Coffee or Tea w/MCT Oil: ○ YES   ○ NO

MEDITATED: ○ YES **LiFT** foundation ○ NO   EXERCISED: ○ YES ○ NO

WHAT I CONSUMED DURING MY 8 HOUR EATING WINDOW:

○ 1 TBSP Braggs Apple Cider Vinegar before brunch

___am BRUNCH   Greens _____   Beans _____   Protein _____

___pm AFTERNOON SNACK _____

○ 1 TBSP Braggs Apple Cider Vinegar before dinner

___pm DINNER Greens _____   Beans _____   Protein _____

___pm EVENING SNACK or BERRIES _____

Alchoholic Beverages? ○ Yes ○ No _____

WATER ⊔ ⊔ ⊔ ⊔ ⊔ ⊔ ⊔ ⊔

CROSS OFF A GLASS EVERY TIME YOU DRINK 8OZ OF WATER

WHAT I CONSUMED *AFTER* MY 8 HOUR EATING WINDOW:

_____

○ I had a phone conversation today with: _____

○ I turned off electronics one hour before bed time at: _____

Today I am especially thankful for: _____

DAILY TRACKING SHEET

WEIGHT

Today I begin again: _____
DATE

🌙 🌙 🌙 🌙 🌙 LAST NIGHT 🌙 🌙 🌙 🌙 🌙

My wakeup goal time was: _____

My actual wakeup time was: _____

Total hours I slept was: _____

SLEEP SCORE

○ I had a very deep sleep
○ I tossed and turned for hours

TODAY

DRANK Coffee or Tea w/MCT Oil: ○ YES   ○ NO

MEDITATED: ○ YES   LiFT foundation   ○ NO | EXERCISED: ○ YES   ○ NO

WHAT I CONSUMED DURING MY 8 HOUR EATING WINDOW:

○ 1 TBSP Braggs Apple Cider Vinegar before brunch

___am BRUNCH   Greens _____   Beans _____   Protein _____

___pm AFTERNOON SNACK _____

○ 1 TBSP Braggs Apple Cider Vinegar before dinner

___pm DINNER   Greens _____   Beans _____   Protein _____

___pm EVENING SNACK or BERRIES _____

Alchoholic Beverages? ○ Yes   ○ No _____

WATER ⬜ ⬜ ⬜ ⬜ ⬜ ⬜ ⬜ ⬜

CROSS OFF A GLASS EVERY TIME YOU DRINK 8OZ OF WATER

WHAT I CONSUMED *AFTER* MY 8 HOUR EATING WINDOW:

○ I had a phone conversation today with: _____

○ I turned off electronics one hour before bed time at: _____

Today I am especially thankful for: _____

DAILY TRACKING SHEET

WEIGHT

Today I begin again: _____
DATE

🌙 🌙 🌙 🌙 🌙 LAST NIGHT 🌙 🌙 🌙 🌙 🌙

My wakeup goal time was: _____

My actual wakeup time was: _____

Total hours I slept was: _____

SLEEP SCORE

○ I had a very deep sleep

○ I tossed and turned for ____ hours

TODAY

DRANK Coffee or Tea w/MCT Oil: ○ YES   ○ NO

MEDITATED: ○ YES LIFT Foundation ○ NO   EXERCISED: ○ YES ○ NO

WHAT I CONSUMED DURING MY 8 HOUR EATING WINDOW:

○ 1 TBSP Braggs Apple Cider Vinegar before brunch

___am BRUNCH   Greens _____   Beans _____   Protein _____

___pm AFTERNOON SNACK _____

○ 1 TBSP Braggs Apple Cider Vinegar before dinner

___pm DINNER Greens _____   Beans _____   Protein _____

___pm EVENING SNACK or BERRIES _____

Alchoholic Beverages? ○ Yes ○ No _____

WATER [ ] [ ] [ ] [ ] [ ] [ ] [ ] [ ]

CROSS OFF A GLASS EVERY TIME YOU DRINK 8OZ OF WATER

WHAT I CONSUMED *AFTER* MY 8 HOUR EATING WINDOW:

_____

○ I had a phone conversation today with: _____

○ I turned off electronics one hour before bed time at: _____

Today I am especially thankful for: _____

<table>
<tr><td>CHEAT DAY?

Y   N</td><td># DAILY TRACKING SHEET

Today I begin again: _____
DATE</td><td>WEIGHT</td></tr>
</table>

🌙 🌙 🌙 🌙 🌙 LAST NIGHT 🌙 🌙 🌙 🌙 🌙

My wakeup goal time was: _____

My actual wakeup time was: _____

Total hours I slept was: _____

SLEEP SCORE

○ I had a very deep sleep

○ I tossed and turned for hours

TODAY

DRANK Coffee or Tea w/MCT Oil: ○ YES   ○ NO

MEDITATED: ○ YES 🦁 LiFT foundation ○ NO   EXERCISED: ○ YES ○ NO

WHAT I CONSUMED DURING MY 8 HOUR EATING WINDOW:

○ 1 TBSP Braggs Apple Cider Vinegar before brunch

___am BRUNCH   Greens _____   Beans _____   Protein _____

___pm AFTERNOON SNACK _____

○ 1 TBSP Braggs Apple Cider Vinegar before dinner

___pm DINNER Greens _____   Beans _____   Protein _____

___pm EVENING SNACK or BERRIES _____

Alchoholic Beverages? ○ Yes ○ No _____

WATER ▢ ▢ ▢ ▢ ▢ ▢ ▢ ▢

CROSS OFF A GLASS EVERY TIME YOU DRINK 8OZ OF WATER

WHAT I CONSUMED *AFTER* MY 8 HOUR EATING WINDOW:

○ I had a phone conversation today with: _____

○ I turned off electronics one hour before bed time at: _____

Today I am especially thankful for: _____

DAILY TRACKING SHEET

WEIGHT

Today I begin again: _____
DATE

🌙 🌙 🌙 🌙 🌙 LAST NIGHT 🌙 🌙 🌙 🌙 🌙

My wakeup goal time was: _____

My actual wakeup time was: _____

Total hours I slept was: _____

SLEEP SCORE

○ I had a very deep sleep

○ I tossed and turned for hours

TODAY

DRANK Coffee or Tea w/MCT Oil: ○ YES   ○ NO

MEDITATED: ○ YES *LIFT foundation* ○ NO | EXERCISED: ○ YES ○ NO

WHAT I CONSUMED DURING MY 8 HOUR EATING WINDOW:

○ 1 TBSP Braggs Apple Cider Vinegar before brunch

___am BRUNCH   Greens _____   Beans _____   Protein _____

___pm AFTERNOON SNACK _____

○ 1 TBSP Braggs Apple Cider Vinegar before dinner

___pm DINNER Greens _____   Beans _____   Protein _____

___pm EVENING SNACK or BERRIES _____

Alchoholic Beverages? ○ Yes ○ No _____

WATER ☐ ☐ ☐ ☐ ☐ ☐ ☐ ☐

CROSS OFF A GLASS EVERY TIME YOU DRINK 8OZ OF WATER

WHAT I CONSUMED *AFTER* MY 8 HOUR EATING WINDOW:

○ I had a phone conversation today with: _____

○ I turned off electronics one hour before bed time at: _____

Today I am especially thankful for: _____

DAY 20! FINISH LINE

CHEAT DAY? Y N

WEIGHT

Today I begin again: _____
DATE

🌙 🌙 🌙 🌙 🌙 LAST NIGHT 🌙 🌙 🌙 🌙 🌙

My wakeup goal time was: _____

My actual wakeup time was: _____

Total hours I slept was: _____

SLEEP SCORE

○ I had a very deep sleep
○ I tossed and turned for hours

TODAY

DRANK Coffee or Tea w/MCT Oil: ○ YES   ○ NO

MEDITATED: ○ YES LiFT foundation ○ NO | EXERCISED: ○ YES ○ NO

WHAT I CONSUMED DURING MY 8 HOUR EATING WINDOW:

○ 1 TBSP Braggs Apple Cider Vinegar before brunch

___am BRUNCH   Greens _____   Beans _____   Protein _____

___pm AFTERNOON SNACK _____

○ 1 TBSP Braggs Apple Cider Vinegar before dinner

___pm DINNER Greens _____   Beans _____   Protein _____

___pm EVENING SNACK or BERRIES _____

Alchoholic Beverages? ○ Yes ○ No _____

WATER ⬜ ⬜ ⬜ ⬜ ⬜ ⬜ ⬜ ⬜

CROSS OFF A GLASS EVERY TIME YOU DRINK 8OZ OF WATER

WHAT I CONSUMED *AFTER* MY 8 HOUR EATING WINDOW:

○ I had a phone conversation today with: _____

○ I turned off electronics one hour before bed time at: _____

Today I am especially thankful for: _____

Final Measurements

Date _____

Neck _____"   o

Arm _____"   o   o - - - - - Chest _____"

                      o - - - - - Belly _____"

Hips _____" - - - o

                o - - - - Thigh _____"

                        Weight _____

                        BP _____

Well Done!

Write your favorite motivational quote in this space:

_____

_____

_____

_____

Notes & Reflections

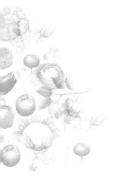

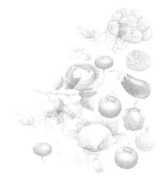

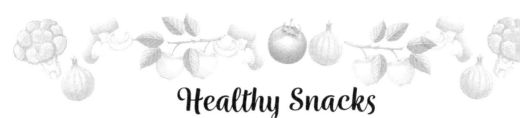

Healthy Snacks

- Walnuts
- Almond Butter
- Cucumbers
- Broccoli
- Carrots

- Apples
- Pears
- Blueberries
- Green Olives
- Hard Boiled Egg

Healthy Snacks I've discovered on my own:

_____

_____

_____

_____

_____

_____

_____

_____

_____

_____

_____

_____

_____

_____

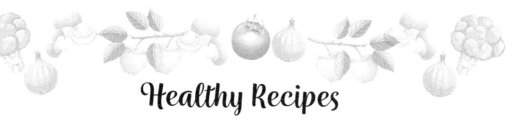

Healthy Recipes

AVOCADO SALAD DRESSING

- 1/2 cup fresh cilantro
- 1/2 cup fresh parsley
- 1/2 jalapeño, seeds removed, and chopped
- 1/2 ripe avocado, halved, pitted, and cut into large chunks
- Zest and juice of 1 lime
- 1 tsp Kosher salt
- 1/2 tsp freshly ground black pepper
- 1/4 cup water
- 1 TBSP extra virgin olive oil
- 1 TBSP hot sauce
- 1/4 cup Greek Yogurt

Directions:

1. Combine & blend in a food processor or high speed blender: cilantro, parsley, jalapeño, avocado, lime zest and juice, salt, and pepper.

2. Once the cilantro and spice mixture is blended together smoothly, add the yogurt, water, olive oil and hot sauce and continue to blend until a smooth, creamy consistency is reached.
Adjust any seasoning to taste. Refrigerate before use.

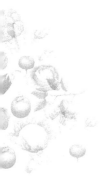
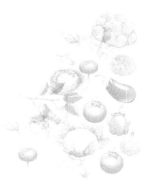

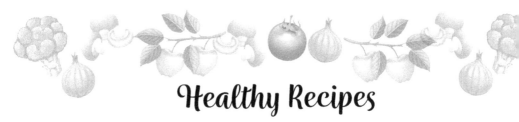

Healthy Recipes

VEGAN CHILI

- 8oz organic tempeh (crumbled)
- 1 large vidalia onion chopped
- 3 cloves garlic chopped
- 2 green peppers chopped
- 8 oz can black beans (drained)
- 8 oz can navy beans or kidney beans (drained)
- 28 oz can whole peeled tomatoes with liquid
- 1 TBSP chili powder
- 1 tsp ground cumin
- 1 tsp black pepper
- 1 tsp crushed red pepper

Optional additions for more healthy yummyness:
- 1 cup cut green beans, • 1 cup chopped carrots,
- 1 TBSP balsamic vinegar, • 1 tsp curry

Directions:

1. Heat oil in large pot over medium heat.
2. Add garlic, onion, and green peppers and sauté until tender.
3. Stir in tempeh crumbles and spices, cook additional 5 minutes.
4. Add tomatoes and beans. Bring mixture to a boil.
5. Reduce heat, cover, and simmer for 20 minutes.

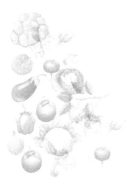
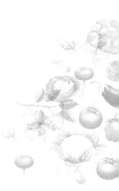

Healthy Recipes

SHRIMP FRIED CAULIFLOWER RICE

- 3 tablespoons vegetable oil, divided
- 8 jumbo shrimp, peeled and de-veined, tails removed
- 2 cups Swiss chard, stems removed and chopped
- Kosher salt and cracked black pepper to taste
- ½ bunch scallions, cut into 1 inch pieces, plus more for garnish
- 3 cloves garlic, sliced
- 2 carrots, diced
- 2 cups cauliflower rice
- 1 cups frozen lima beans, thawed
- 3 tablespoons grated ginger
- 3 tablespoons tamari

Optional additions for more healthy yummyness: • Lime wedges,
• ¼ teaspoon red pepper flakes, • Toasted and crushed peanuts

Directions:

1. Heat a large non-stick skillet over medium high heat and add 1TBSP of the oil. Season the shrimp with S&P and once the pan is very hot, add the shrimp. Cook for 3 to 4 min. until bright pink. Remove to a plate and set aside.

2. Add another TBSP of the oil and cook the chard until wilted, about 3 minutes. Season with salt and remove from the pan with any of its liquid and set aside on a paper towel lined plate to remove excess moisture.

3. Add the remaining oil to the pan and add in the scallion, cook for 2 to 3 minutes. Add in the garlic and the carrots and season with salt. Add in the cauliflower rice and toss to combine and then leave undisturbed for 1 to 2 minutes to get a little crispy. Toss again and let cook for an additional minute undisturbed. Stir in the lima beans.

4. In a small bowl, combine the ginger, tamari, and pepper flake if using.

5. Add the shrimp and the chard back to the pan and toss to combine. Pour in the tamari to coat all of the veggies and shrimp. Spoon the fried "rice" into two bowls and top with remaining scallions, crushed peanuts, and lime.

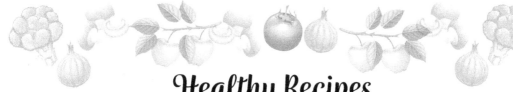

Healthy Recipes

SUPER GREEN SALMON BOWL

- 2, 4 ounce salmon filetts, boneless and skinless
- 3 TBSP vegetable oil, divided
- 2 cups shelled edamame, thawed
- Kosher salt and freshly cracked black pepper, to taste
- 2 TBSP toasted sesame oil
- 2 lbs baby spinach
- 2 cloves garlic, minced
- 1 inch piece of ginger, peeled and grated
- 1 cucumber, thinly sliced
- 4 radishes, thinly sliced
- 2 TBSP rice wine vinegar
- 2 scallions, thinly sliced
- ½ an avocado, sliced
- Optional: 1 TBSP tamari, & Lime wedges for garnish

Directions:

1. Preheat the oven to 350 degrees F

2. Place the salmon onto one side of a sheet pan and drizzle with 1 ½ TBSP vegetable oil. Season with S&P.

3. Place the edamame in a small bowl and add the remaining 1 ½ TBSP oil. Toss to combine and add to the other side of the sheet pan. Place into the oven and cook for 6 to 8 minutes. Set aside.

4. Place a medium non-stick skillet over medium heat and add in the sesame oil and the garlic. Add the spinach and season with salt. Toss to wilt and add in the ginger. Remove from the heat.

5. Place the cucumbers, radish, scallion, the rice vinegar into a bowl. Season with salt and set aside.

6. To build the bowl, place half of the edamame into a bowl and top with half of the spinach. Place a piece of salmon on top and place half of the cucumber-carrot-radish mixture next to that. Drizzle with tamari if using and garnish with, avocado slices, and lime wedge. Repeat with the remaining ingredients.

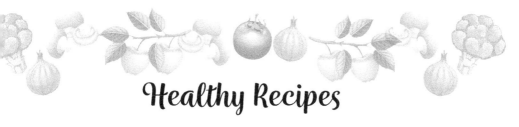

Healthy Recipes

SHEET PAN SQUASH with CHICKPEAS, BROCCOLI RABE and WALNUT PESTO

- 2 cups cubed butternut squash
- 2 TBSP olive oil, divided
- 1 cup chickpeas, drained and rinsed
- 1 bunch broccoli rabe
- ½ onion, sliced
- Kosher salt and cracked black pepper to taste
- 2 eggs
- 1 TBSP white vinegar

For the pesto:
- ½ cup walnuts
- 1 clove garlic
- ¼ cup grated parmesan cheese
- 1 bunch basil, leaves only
- Zest and juice of 1 lemon
- ¼ cup olive oil

Poached Egg:
Fill a small sauce pot with water and vinegar and bring to a simmer. Stir with a slotted spoon and place the eggs into the water. Cook until the whites have set but the yolks are still runny, about 4 minutes.

Directions:

1. Preheat the oven to 400 degrees F

2. Place the squash onto a sheet pan and drizzle with half of the olive oil. Season with S&P. Place in the oven and roast for 15 minutes or until tender, stirring halfway through.

3. Place the broccoli and the chickpeas on a sheet pan with the sliced onion and season with S&P. Place into the oven for 15 minutes, stirring halfway through.

4. While the vegetables cook, make the pesto by placing all of the ingredients into the food processor except for the oil and pulsing to combine. With the motor running stream in the olive oil until smooth.

5. Divide the chickpeas and broccoli evenly between two bowls. Place the squash into a separate bowl and toss with the pesto. Place over the broccoli and the chickpeas. Top with the poached egg.

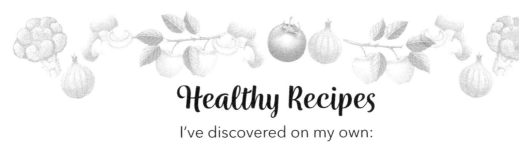

Healthy Recipes

I've discovered on my own:

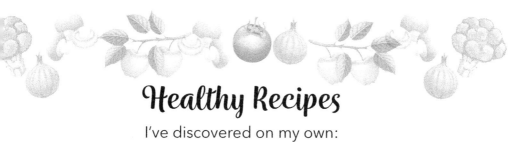

Healthy Recipes

I've discovered on my own:

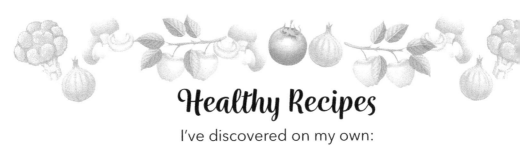

Healthy Recipes

I've discovered on my own:

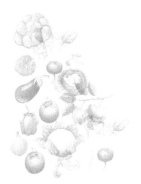

Healthy Recipes

I've discovered on my own:

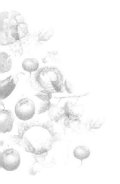

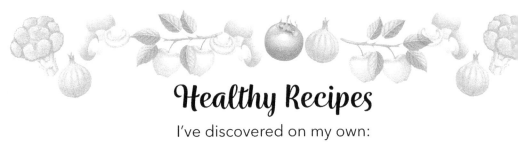

Healthy Recipes

I've discovered on my own:

Healthy Recipes

I've discovered on my own:

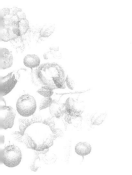

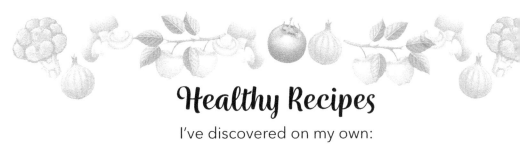

Healthy Recipes

I've discovered on my own:

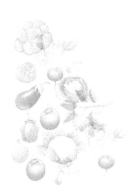

Before Photo

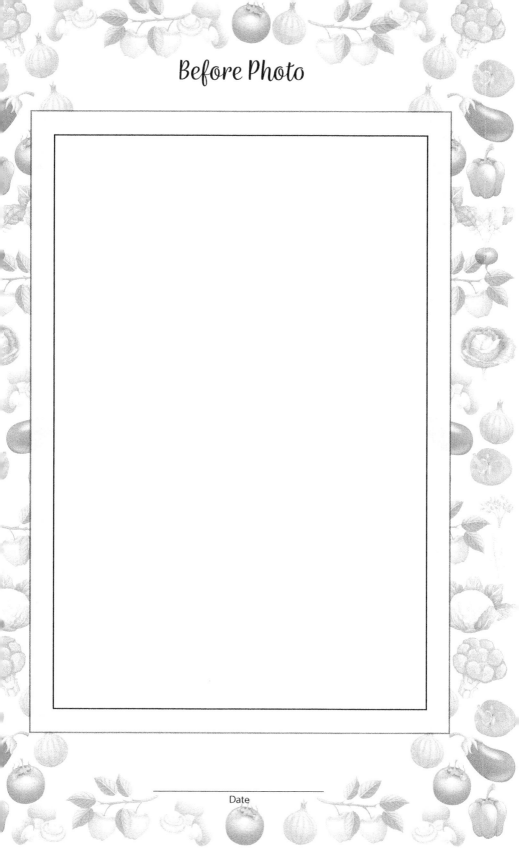

Date

After Photo

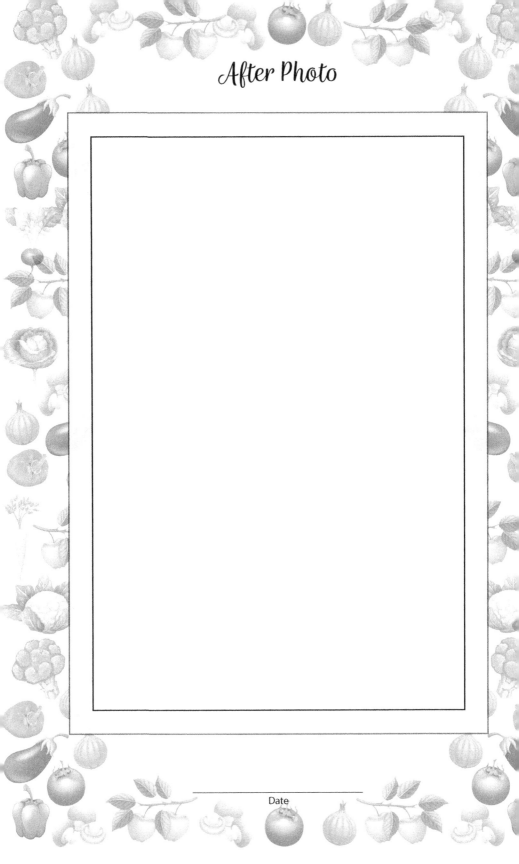

_____
Date

Notes & Reflections

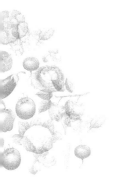

Postive Affirmations

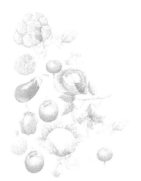

Bonus Section

Want to keep going? Or start again?

This section gives you 20 add'l days.

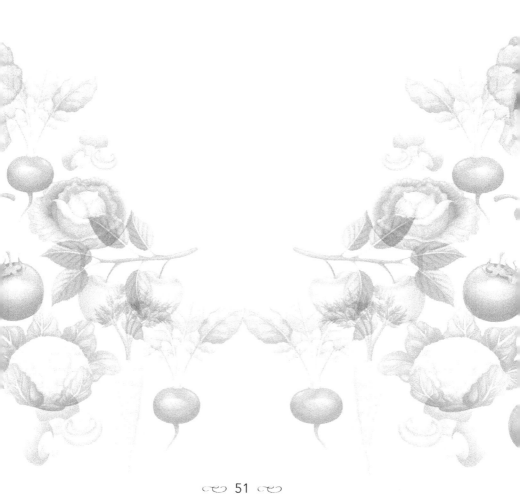

CHEAT DAY?	# DAILY TRACKING SHEET	WEIGHT
Y N	Today I begin again: _____ DATE	

My wakeup goal time was: _____

My actual wakeup time was: _____

Total hours I slept was: _____

SLEEP SCORE

○ I had a very deep sleep

○ I tossed and turned for hours

TODAY

DRANK Coffee or Tea w/MCT Oil: ○ YES   ○ NO

MEDITATED: ○ YES LiFT foundation ○ NO   EXERCISED: ○ YES ○ NO

WHAT I CONSUMED DURING MY 8 HOUR EATING WINDOW:

○ 1 TBSP Braggs Apple Cider Vinegar before brunch

___am BRUNCH   Greens _____   Beans _____   Protein _____

___pm AFTERNOON SNACK _____

○ 1 TBSP Braggs Apple Cider Vinegar before dinner

___pm DINNER Greens _____   Beans _____   Protein _____

___pm EVENING SNACK or BERRIES _____

Alchoholic Beverages? ○ Yes ○ No _____

WATER ☐ ☐ ☐ ☐ ☐ ☐ ☐ ☐

CROSS OFF A GLASS EVERY TIME YOU DRINK 8OZ OF WATER

WHAT I CONSUMED *AFTER* MY 8 HOUR EATING WINDOW:

○ I had a phone conversation today with: _____

○ I turned off electronics one hour before bed time at: _____

Today I am especially thankful for:_____

DAILY TRACKING SHEET

Today I begin again: _____
DATE

🌙🌙🌙🌙🌙 LAST NIGHT 🌙🌙🌙🌙🌙

My wakeup goal time was: _____

My actual wakeup time was: _____

Total hours I slept was: _____

SLEEP SCORE

○ I had a very deep sleep
○ I tossed and turned for hours

TODAY

DRANK Coffee or Tea w/MCT Oil: ○ YES   ○ NO

MEDITATED: ○ YES ⚡LiFT foundation ○ NO   EXERCISED: ○ YES ○ NO

WHAT I CONSUMED DURING MY 8 HOUR EATING WINDOW:

○ 1 TBSP Braggs Apple Cider Vinegar before brunch

___am BRUNCH   Greens _____   Beans _____   Protein _____

___pm AFTERNOON SNACK _____

○ 1 TBSP Braggs Apple Cider Vinegar before dinner

___pm DINNER Greens _____   Beans _____   Protein _____

___pm EVENING SNACK or BERRIES _____

Alchoholic Beverages? ○ Yes ○ No _____

WATER ⬚⬚⬚⬚⬚⬚⬚⬚

CROSS OFF A GLASS EVERY TIME YOU DRINK 8OZ OF WATER

WHAT I CONSUMED *AFTER* MY 8 HOUR EATING WINDOW:

○ I had a phone conversation today with: _____

○ I turned off electronics one hour before bed time at: _____

Today I am especially thankful for: _____

DAILY TRACKING SHEET

WEIGHT

Today I begin again: _____
DATE

🌙 🌙 🌙 🌙 🌙 LAST NIGHT 🌙 🌙 🌙 🌙 🌙

My wakeup goal time was: _____

My actual wakeup time was: _____

Total hours I slept was: _____

SLEEP SCORE

○ I had a very deep sleep

○ I tossed and turned for hours

TODAY

DRANK Coffee or Tea w/MCT Oil: ○ YES   ○ NO

MEDITATED: ○ YES LIFT Foundation ○ NO | EXERCISED: ○ YES ○ NO

WHAT I CONSUMED DURING MY 8 HOUR EATING WINDOW:

○ 1 TBSP Braggs Apple Cider Vinegar before brunch

___am BRUNCH   Greens _____   Beans _____   Protein _____

___pm AFTERNOON SNACK _____

○ 1 TBSP Braggs Apple Cider Vinegar before dinner

___pm DINNER Greens _____   Beans _____   Protein _____

___pm EVENING SNACK or BERRIES _____

Alchoholic Beverages? ○ Yes ○ No _____

WATER ☐ ☐ ☐ ☐ ☐ ☐ ☐ ☐

CROSS OFF A GLASS EVERY TIME YOU DRINK 8OZ OF WATER

WHAT I CONSUMED *AFTER* MY 8 HOUR EATING WINDOW:

○ I had a phone conversation today with: _____

○ I turned off electronics one hour before bed time at: _____

Today I am especially thankful for: _____

DAILY TRACKING SHEET

Today I begin again: _____
DATE

🌙 🌙 🌙 🌙 🌙 LAST NIGHT 🌙 🌙 🌙 🌙 🌙

My wakeup goal time was: _____	SLEEP SCORE	○ I had a very deep sleep
My actual wakeup time was: _____		○ I tossed and turned for hours
Total hours I slept was: _____		

TODAY

DRANK Coffee or Tea w/MCT Oil: ○ YES   ○ NO

MEDITATED: ○ YES _LIFT_ foundation ○ NO | EXERCISED: ○ YES ○ NO

WHAT I CONSUMED DURING MY 8 HOUR EATING WINDOW:

○ 1 TBSP Braggs Apple Cider Vinegar before brunch

___am BRUNCH   Greens _____   Beans _____   Protein _____

___pm AFTERNOON SNACK _____

○ 1 TBSP Braggs Apple Cider Vinegar before dinner

___pm DINNER Greens _____   Beans _____   Protein _____

___pm EVENING SNACK or BERRIES _____

Alchoholic Beverages? ○ Yes ○ No _____

WATER ▢ ▢ ▢ ▢ ▢ ▢ ▢ ▢

CROSS OFF A GLASS EVERY TIME YOU DRINK 8OZ OF WATER

WHAT I CONSUMED *AFTER* MY 8 HOUR EATING WINDOW:

○ I had a phone conversation today with: _____

○ I turned off electronics one hour before bed time at: _____

Today I am especially thankful for: _____

DAILY TRACKING SHEET

Today I begin again: _____
DATE

🌙 🌙 🌙 🌙 🌙 LAST NIGHT 🌙 🌙 🌙 🌙 🌙

My wakeup goal time was: _____

My actual wakeup time was: _____

Total hours I slept was: _____

SLEEP SCORE	○ I had a very deep sleep
	○ I tossed and turned for hours

TODAY

DRANK Coffee or Tea w/MCT Oil: ○ YES   ○ NO

MEDITATED: ○ YES ⚡LiFT foundation ○ NO | EXERCISED: ○ YES ○ NO

WHAT I CONSUMED DURING MY 8 HOUR EATING WINDOW:

○ 1 TBSP Braggs Apple Cider Vinegar before brunch

___am BRUNCH   Greens _____   Beans _____   Protein _____

___pm AFTERNOON SNACK _____

○ 1 TBSP Braggs Apple Cider Vinegar before dinner

___pm DINNER Greens _____   Beans _____   Protein _____

___pm EVENING SNACK or BERRIES _____

Alchoholic Beverages? ○ Yes ○ No _____

WATER ☐ ☐ ☐ ☐ ☐ ☐ ☐ ☐

CROSS OFF A GLASS EVERY TIME YOU DRINK 8OZ OF WATER

WHAT I CONSUMED *AFTER* MY 8 HOUR EATING WINDOW:

○ I had a phone conversation today with: _____

○ I turned off electronics one hour before bed time at: _____

Today I am especially thankful for: _____

DAILY TRACKING SHEET

WEIGHT

Today I begin again: _____
DATE

LAST NIGHT

My wakeup goal time was: _____

My actual wakeup time was: _____

Total hours I slept was: _____

SLEEP SCORE

O I had a very deep sleep

O I tossed and turned for hours

TODAY

DRANK Coffee or Tea w/MCT Oil: O YES   O NO

MEDITATED: O YES LIFT foundation O NO | EXERCISED: O YES O NO

WHAT I CONSUMED DURING MY 8 HOUR EATING WINDOW:

O 1 TBSP Braggs Apple Cider Vinegar before brunch

___am BRUNCH   Greens _____   Beans _____   Protein _____

___pm AFTERNOON SNACK _____

O 1 TBSP Braggs Apple Cider Vinegar before dinner

___pm DINNER Greens _____   Beans _____   Protein _____

___pm EVENING SNACK or BERRIES _____

Alchoholic Beverages? O Yes O No _____

WATER ⬚ ⬚ ⬚ ⬚ ⬚ ⬚ ⬚ ⬚

CROSS OFF A GLASS EVERY TIME YOU DRINK 8OZ OF WATER

WHAT I CONSUMED *AFTER* MY 8 HOUR EATING WINDOW:

O I had a phone conversation today with: _____

O I turned off electronics one hour before bed time at: _____

Today I am especially thankful for: _____

DAILY TRACKING SHEET

Today I begin again: _____
DATE

🌙 🌙 🌙 🌙 🌙 LAST NIGHT 🌙 🌙 🌙 🌙 🌙

My wakeup goal time was: _____

My actual wakeup time was: _____

Total hours I slept was: _____

SLEEP SCORE

○ I had a very deep sleep

○ I tossed and turned for hours

TODAY

DRANK Coffee or Tea w/MCT Oil: ○ YES   ○ NO

MEDITATED: ○ YES LiFT foundation ○ NO | EXERCISED: ○ YES ○ NO

WHAT I CONSUMED DURING MY 8 HOUR EATING WINDOW:

○ 1 TBSP Braggs Apple Cider Vinegar before brunch

___am BRUNCH   Greens _____   Beans _____   Protein _____

___pm AFTERNOON SNACK _____

○ 1 TBSP Braggs Apple Cider Vinegar before dinner

___pm DINNER Greens _____   Beans _____   Protein _____

___pm EVENING SNACK or BERRIES _____

Alchoholic Beverages? ○ Yes ○ No _____

WATER ▯ ▯ ▯ ▯ ▯ ▯ ▯ ▯

CROSS OFF A GLASS EVERY TIME YOU DRINK 8OZ OF WATER

WHAT I CONSUMED *AFTER* MY 8 HOUR EATING WINDOW:

○ I had a phone conversation today with: _____

○ I turned off electronics one hour before bed time at: _____

Today I am especially thankful for: _____

DAILY TRACKING SHEET

Today I begin again: _____
DATE

LAST NIGHT

My wakeup goal time was: _____

My actual wakeup time was: _____

Total hours I slept was: _____

SLEEP SCORE

○ I had a very deep sleep

○ I tossed and turned for hours

TODAY

DRANK Coffee or Tea w/MCT Oil: ○ YES   ○ NO

MEDITATED: ○ YES LiFT foundation ○ NO | EXERCISED: ○ YES ○ NO

WHAT I CONSUMED DURING MY 8 HOUR EATING WINDOW:

○ 1 TBSP Braggs Apple Cider Vinegar before brunch

___am BRUNCH   Greens _____   Beans _____   Protein _____

___pm AFTERNOON SNACK _____

○ 1 TBSP Braggs Apple Cider Vinegar before dinner

___pm DINNER Greens _____   Beans _____   Protein _____

___pm EVENING SNACK or BERRIES _____

Alchoholic Beverages? ○ Yes ○ No _____

WATER ☐ ☐ ☐ ☐ ☐ ☐ ☐ ☐

CROSS OFF A GLASS EVERY TIME YOU DRINK 8OZ OF WATER

WHAT I CONSUMED AFTER MY 8 HOUR EATING WINDOW:

○ I had a phone conversation today with: _____

○ I turned off electronics one hour before bed time at: _____

Today I am especially thankful for: _____

CHEAT DAY?	# DAILY TRACKING SHEET	WEIGHT
Y N	Today I begin again: _____ DATE	

🌙 🌙 🌙 🌙 🌙 **LAST NIGHT** 🌙 🌙 🌙 🌙 🌙

My wakeup goal time was: _____ My actual wakeup time was: _____ Total hours I slept was: _____	SLEEP SCORE	◯ I had a very deep sleep ◯ I tossed and turned for hours

TODAY

DRANK Coffee or Tea w/MCT Oil: ◯ YES ◯ NO

MEDITATED: ◯ YES 🐺 LiFT Foundation ◯ NO | EXERCISED: ◯ YES ◯ NO

WHAT I CONSUMED DURING MY 8 HOUR EATING WINDOW:

◯ 1 TBSP Braggs Apple Cider Vinegar before brunch

___am BRUNCH   Greens _____   Beans _____   Protein _____

___pm AFTERNOON SNACK _____

◯ 1 TBSP Braggs Apple Cider Vinegar before dinner

___pm DINNER Greens _____   Beans _____   Protein _____

___pm EVENING SNACK or BERRIES _____

Alchoholic Beverages? ◯ Yes ◯ No _____

WATER ☐ ☐ ☐ ☐ ☐ ☐ ☐ ☐

CROSS OFF A GLASS EVERY TIME YOU DRINK 8OZ OF WATER

WHAT I CONSUMED *AFTER* MY 8 HOUR EATING WINDOW:

◯ I had a phone conversation today with: _____

◯ I turned off electronics one hour before bed time at: _____

Today I am especially thankful for: _____

DAILY TRACKING SHEET

Today I begin again: _____
DATE

WEIGHT

LAST NIGHT

My wakeup goal time was: _____

My actual wakeup time was: _____

Total hours I slept was: _____

SLEEP SCORE

○ I had a very deep sleep

○ I tossed and turned for hours

TODAY

DRANK Coffee or Tea w/MCT Oil: ○ YES   ○ NO

MEDITATED: ○ YES ⚡LiFT foundation ○ NO | EXERCISED: ○ YES ○ NO

WHAT I CONSUMED DURING MY 8 HOUR EATING WINDOW:

○ 1 TBSP Braggs Apple Cider Vinegar before brunch

___am BRUNCH   Greens _____   Beans _____   Protein _____

___pm AFTERNOON SNACK _____

○ 1 TBSP Braggs Apple Cider Vinegar before dinner

___pm DINNER Greens _____   Beans _____   Protein _____

___pm EVENING SNACK or BERRIES _____

Alchoholic Beverages? ○ Yes   ○ No _____

WATER ⬜ ⬜ ⬜ ⬜ ⬜ ⬜ ⬜ ⬜

CROSS OFF A GLASS EVERY TIME YOU DRINK 8OZ OF WATER

WHAT I CONSUMED AFTER MY 8 HOUR EATING WINDOW:

○ I had a phone conversation today with: _____

○ I turned off electronics one hour before bed time at: _____

Today I am especially thankful for: _____

LAST NIGHT

My wakeup goal time was: _____

My actual wakeup time was: _____

Total hours I slept was: _____

SLEEP SCORE

○ I had a very deep sleep

○ I tossed and turned for hours

TODAY

DRANK Coffee or Tea w/MCT Oil: ○ YES   ○ NO

MEDITATED: ○ YES LiFT foundation ○ NO | EXERCISED: ○ YES ○ NO

WHAT I CONSUMED DURING MY 8 HOUR EATING WINDOW:

○ 1 TBSP Braggs Apple Cider Vinegar before brunch

___am BRUNCH   Greens _____   Beans _____   Protein _____

___pm AFTERNOON SNACK _____

○ 1 TBSP Braggs Apple Cider Vinegar before dinner

___pm DINNER Greens _____   Beans _____   Protein _____

___pm EVENING SNACK or BERRIES _____

Alchoholic Beverages? ○ Yes ○ No _____

WATER ☐ ☐ ☐ ☐ ☐ ☐ ☐ ☐

CROSS OFF A GLASS EVERY TIME YOU DRINK 8OZ OF WATER

WHAT I CONSUMED AFTER MY 8 HOUR EATING WINDOW:

○ I had a phone conversation today with: _____

○ I turned off electronics one hour before bed time at: _____

Today I am especially thankful for: _____

CHEAT DAY?
Y   N

DAILY TRACKING SHEET

Today I begin again: _____
DATE

WEIGHT

🌙 🌙 🌙 🌙 🌙 LAST NIGHT 🌙 🌙 🌙 🌙 🌙

My wakeup goal time was: _____

My actual wakeup time was: _____

Total hours I slept was: _____

SLEEP SCORE

○ I had a very deep sleep

○ I tossed and turned for hours

TODAY

DRANK Coffee or Tea w/MCT Oil: ○ YES   ○ NO

MEDITATED: ○ YES 🦅LiFT foundation   ○ NO | EXERCISED: ○ YES   ○ NO

WHAT I CONSUMED DURING MY 8 HOUR EATING WINDOW:

○ 1 TBSP Braggs Apple Cider Vinegar before brunch

___am BRUNCH   Greens _____   Beans _____   Protein _____

___pm AFTERNOON SNACK _____

○ 1 TBSP Braggs Apple Cider Vinegar before dinner

___pm DINNER Greens _____   Beans _____   Protein _____

___pm EVENING SNACK or BERRIES _____

Alchoholic Beverages? ○ Yes ○ No _____

WATER ☐ ☐ ☐ ☐ ☐ ☐ ☐ ☐

CROSS OFF A GLASS EVERY TIME YOU DRINK 8OZ OF WATER

WHAT I CONSUMED AFTER MY 8 HOUR EATING WINDOW:

○ I had a phone conversation today with: _____

○ I turned off electronics one hour before bed time at: _____

Today I am especially thankful for: _____

DAILY TRACKING SHEET

CHEAT DAY?

Y   N

Today I begin again: _____
DATE

WEIGHT

LAST NIGHT

My wakeup goal time was: _____

My actual wakeup time was: _____

Total hours I slept was: _____

SLEEP SCORE

○ I had a very deep sleep

○ I tossed and turned for hours

TODAY

DRANK Coffee or Tea w/MCT Oil: ○ YES   ○ NO

MEDITATED: ○ YES ⚡LiFT ○ NO | EXERCISED: ○ YES ○ NO

WHAT I CONSUMED DURING MY 8 HOUR EATING WINDOW:

○ 1 TBSP Braggs Apple Cider Vinegar before brunch

___am BRUNCH   Greens _____   Beans _____   Protein _____

___pm AFTERNOON SNACK _____

○ 1 TBSP Braggs Apple Cider Vinegar before dinner

___pm DINNER Greens _____   Beans _____   Protein _____

___pm EVENING SNACK or BERRIES _____

Alchoholic Beverages? ○ Yes ○ No _____

WATER ☐ ☐ ☐ ☐ ☐ ☐ ☐ ☐

CROSS OFF A GLASS EVERY TIME YOU DRINK 8OZ OF WATER

WHAT I CONSUMED AFTER MY 8 HOUR EATING WINDOW:

○ I had a phone conversation today with: _____

○ I turned off electronics one hour before bed time at: _____

Today I am especially thankful for: _____

DAILY TRACKING SHEET

WEIGHT

Today I begin again: _____
DATE

LAST NIGHT

My wakeup goal time was: _____

My actual wakeup time was: _____

Total hours I slept was: _____

SLEEP SCORE

○ I had a very deep sleep

○ I tossed and turned for hours

TODAY

DRANK Coffee or Tea w/MCT Oil: ○ YES   ○ NO

MEDITATED: ○ YES LiFT foundation ○ NO | EXERCISED: ○ YES ○ NO

WHAT I CONSUMED DURING MY 8 HOUR EATING WINDOW:

○ 1 TBSP Braggs Apple Cider Vinegar before brunch

___am **BRUNCH**   Greens _____   Beans _____   Protein _____

___pm **AFTERNOON SNACK** _____

○ 1 TBSP Braggs Apple Cider Vinegar before dinner

___pm **DINNER** Greens _____   Beans _____   Protein _____

___pm **EVENING SNACK or BERRIES** _____

Alchoholic Beverages? ○ Yes   ○ No _____

WATER ⬜ ⬜ ⬜ ⬜ ⬜ ⬜ ⬜ ⬜

CROSS OFF A GLASS EVERY TIME YOU DRINK 8OZ OF WATER

WHAT I CONSUMED *AFTER* MY 8 HOUR EATING WINDOW:

_____

○ I had a phone conversation today with: _____

○ I turned off electronics one hour before bed time at: _____

Today I am especially thankful for: _____

DAILY TRACKING SHEET

Today I begin again: _____
DATE

🌙 🌙 🌙 🌙 🌙 LAST NIGHT 🌙 🌙 🌙 🌙 🌙

My wakeup goal time was: _____

My actual wakeup time was: _____

Total hours I slept was: _____

SLEEP SCORE	○ I had a very deep sleep ○ I tossed and turned for hours

TODAY

DRANK Coffee or Tea w/MCT Oil: ○ YES ○ NO

MEDITATED: ○ YES LIFT foundation ○ NO | EXERCISED: ○ YES ○ NO

WHAT I CONSUMED DURING MY 8 HOUR EATING WINDOW:

○ 1 TBSP Braggs Apple Cider Vinegar before brunch

___am BRUNCH   Greens _____   Beans _____   Protein _____

___pm AFTERNOON SNACK _____

○ 1 TBSP Braggs Apple Cider Vinegar before dinner

___pm DINNER Greens _____   Beans _____   Protein _____

___pm EVENING SNACK or BERRIES _____

Alchoholic Beverages? ○ Yes ○ No _____

WATER ☐ ☐ ☐ ☐ ☐ ☐ ☐

CROSS OFF A GLASS EVERY TIME YOU DRINK 8OZ OF WATER

WHAT I CONSUMED AFTER MY 8 HOUR EATING WINDOW:

○ I had a phone conversation today with: _____

○ I turned off electronics one hour before bed time at: _____

Today I am especially thankful for: _____

DAILY TRACKING SHEET

Today I begin again: _____
DATE

🌙 🌙 🌙 🌙 🌙 LAST NIGHT 🌙 🌙 🌙 🌙 🌙

My wakeup goal time was: _____

My actual wakeup time was: _____

Total hours I slept was: _____

SLEEP SCORE

○ I had a very deep sleep

○ I tossed and turned for hours

TODAY

DRANK Coffee or Tea w/MCT Oil: ○ YES   ○ NO

MEDITATED: ○ YES 🦅LIFT ○ NO | EXERCISED: ○ YES   ○ NO
foundation

WHAT I CONSUMED DURING MY 8 HOUR EATING WINDOW:

○ 1 TBSP Braggs Apple Cider Vinegar before brunch

___am BRUNCH   Greens _____   Beans _____   Protein _____

___pm AFTERNOON SNACK _____

○ 1 TBSP Braggs Apple Cider Vinegar before dinner

___pm DINNER Greens _____   Beans _____   Protein _____

___pm EVENING SNACK or BERRIES _____

Alchoholic Beverages? ○ Yes   ○ No _____

WATER [ ] [ ] [ ] [ ] [ ] [ ] [ ] [ ]

CROSS OFF A GLASS EVERY TIME YOU DRINK 8OZ OF WATER

WHAT I CONSUMED *AFTER* MY 8 HOUR EATING WINDOW:

○ I had a phone conversation today with: _____

○ I turned off electronics one hour before bed time at: _____

Today I am especially thankful for: _____

CHEAT DAY?	# DAILY TRACKING SHEET	WEIGHT
Y N	Today I begin again: _____ DATE	

LAST NIGHT

My wakeup goal time was: _____

My actual wakeup time was: _____

Total hours I slept was: _____

SLEEP SCORE

○ I had a very deep sleep

○ I tossed and turned for hours

TODAY

DRANK Coffee or Tea w/MCT Oil: ○ YES   ○ NO

MEDITATED: ○ YES ⚡LiFT Foundation ○ NO | EXERCISED: ○ YES ○ NO

WHAT I CONSUMED DURING MY 8 HOUR EATING WINDOW:

○ 1 TBSP Braggs Apple Cider Vinegar before brunch

___am BRUNCH   Greens _____   Beans _____   Protein _____

___pm AFTERNOON SNACK _____

○ 1 TBSP Braggs Apple Cider Vinegar before dinner

___pm DINNER Greens _____   Beans _____   Protein _____

___pm EVENING SNACK or BERRIES _____

Alchoholic Beverages? ○ Yes ○ No _____

WATER ⬜ ⬜ ⬜ ⬜ ⬜ ⬜ ⬜ ⬜

CROSS OFF A GLASS EVERY TIME YOU DRINK 8OZ OF WATER

WHAT I CONSUMED *AFTER* MY 8 HOUR EATING WINDOW:

○ I had a phone conversation today with: _____

○ I turned off electronics one hour before bed time at: _____

Today I am especially thankful for: _____

DAILY TRACKING SHEET

Today I begin again: _____
DATE

LAST NIGHT

My wakeup goal time was: _____

My actual wakeup time was: _____

Total hours I slept was: _____

SLEEP SCORE

○ I had a very deep sleep

○ I tossed and turned for hours

TODAY

DRANK Coffee or Tea w/MCT Oil: ○ YES   ○ NO

MEDITATED: ○ YES LiFT foundation   ○ NO | EXERCISED: ○ YES   ○ NO

WHAT I CONSUMED DURING MY 8 HOUR EATING WINDOW:

○ 1 TBSP Braggs Apple Cider Vinegar before brunch

___am BRUNCH   Greens _____   Beans _____   Protein _____

___pm AFTERNOON SNACK _____

○ 1 TBSP Braggs Apple Cider Vinegar before dinner

___pm DINNER Greens _____   Beans _____   Protein _____

___pm EVENING SNACK or BERRIES _____

Alchoholic Beverages? ○ Yes   ○ No _____

WATER ⊔ ⊔ ⊔ ⊔ ⊔ ⊔ ⊔ ⊔

CROSS OFF A GLASS EVERY TIME YOU DRINK 8OZ OF WATER

WHAT I CONSUMED *AFTER* MY 8 HOUR EATING WINDOW:

○ I had a phone conversation today with: _____

○ I turned off electronics one hour before bed time at: _____

Today I am especially thankful for: _____

Today I begin again: _____

DATE

🌙 🌙 🌙 🌙 🌙   LAST NIGHT   🌙 🌙 🌙 🌙 🌙

My wakeup goal time was: _____

My actual wakeup time was: _____

Total hours I slept was: _____

SLEEP SCORE

○ I had a very deep sleep

○ I tossed and turned for hours

TODAY

DRANK Coffee or Tea w/MCT Oil: ○ YES ○ NO

MEDITATED: ○ YES 𝕷iFT ○ NO   EXERCISED: ○ YES ○ NO

WHAT I CONSUMED DURING MY 8 HOUR EATING WINDOW:

○ 1 TBSP Braggs Apple Cider Vinegar before brunch

___am BRUNCH   Greens _____   Beans _____   Protein _____

___pm AFTERNOON SNACK _____

○ 1 TBSP Braggs Apple Cider Vinegar before dinner

___pm DINNER   Greens _____   Beans _____   Protein _____

___pm EVENING SNACK or BERRIES _____

Alchoholic Beverages? ○ Yes ○ No _____

WATER 🥛 🥛 🥛 🥛 🥛 🥛 🥛 🥛

CROSS OFF A GLASS EVERY TIME YOU DRINK 8OZ OF WATER

WHAT I CONSUMED *AFTER* MY 8 HOUR EATING WINDOW:

○ I had a phone conversation today with: _____

○ I turned off electronics one hour before bed time at: _____

Today I am especially thankful for: _____

DAILY TRACKING SHEET

<table>
<tr><td>CHEAT
DAY?

Y   N</td><td>Today I begin again: _____
 DATE </td><td>WEIGHT</td></tr>
</table>

LAST NIGHT

My wakeup goal time was: _____

My actual wakeup time was: _____

Total hours I slept was: _____

SLEEP SCORE

○ I had a very deep sleep

○ I tossed and turned for hours

TODAY

DRANK Coffee or Tea w/MCT Oil: ○ YES   ○ NO

MEDITATED: ○ YES LiFT foundation ○ NO | EXERCISED: ○ YES ○ NO

WHAT I CONSUMED DURING MY 8 HOUR EATING WINDOW:

○ 1 TBSP Braggs Apple Cider Vinegar before brunch

___am BRUNCH   Greens _____   Beans _____   Protein _____

___pm AFTERNOON SNACK _____

○ 1 TBSP Braggs Apple Cider Vinegar before dinner

___pm DINNER Greens _____   Beans _____   Protein _____

___pm EVENING SNACK or BERRIES _____

Alchoholic Beverages? ○ Yes ○ No _____

WATER ⊔ ⊔ ⊔ ⊔ ⊔ ⊔ ⊔ ⊔

CROSS OFF A GLASS EVERY TIME YOU DRINK 8OZ OF WATER

WHAT I CONSUMED *AFTER* MY 8 HOUR EATING WINDOW:

○ I had a phone conversation today with: _____

○ I turned off electronics one hour before bed time at: _____

Today I am especially thankful for: _____

Measurements

Date _____

Neck _____ "

Arm _____ "

Chest _____ "

Belly _____ "

Hips _____ "

Thigh _____ "

Weight _____

BP _____

When you feel like

QUITTING.

Think about

WHY

you started.

Bonus System 20 Snacks

2g. lean deli meat - turkey, or chicken
3g. canned tuna
1 hard boiled egg
14 walnut halves
1/2 c Roasted pumpkin seeds
1/4 c almonds
1/2 med. avocado
1/2 c. Edamame
1/2 c. berries
1 mandarin
1/2 c unsweetened coconut flakes
1g. 70% dark chocolate
10 green olives
8g. bone broth
1/2 c. kale chips
15 cheese chips
1 pickle
6g unsweetened, plain whole milk yogurt
6g greek yogurt

Low CARb cheat sheet

Sweet Combos

½ c. cottage Cheese + 1 tbsp cocoa nibs + hand full of Raspberries

1 med. apple, sliced + 1 TBSP peanut butter

3.5 oz cantaloupe + 2 tbsp. whipped heavy cream

1 small pear + 3.5 oz ricotta cheese

2 tbs chia seeds + ½ c. milk + 1 tsp. Vanilla stevia

SAVory Pairings

½ red pepper + 2 z. guac

½ cucumber + 2 tbsp hummus

1 c. broccoli + 1 tbsp tahini

1 tomato, sliced + 2 z. mozzarella cheese

1 handfull baby CARRots + 2 tbsp blue cheese

1 c. baked Zucchini chips + paprika & sea salt

6 flax seed Crackers + 1 z. cheese

Shopping list

Protein
Lean deli meat Chicken or turkey

Eggs

Tuna

Shrimp

Chicken thighs

Salmon

Tofu

ground Turkey

ground Chicken

Beans
Chick peas

Lima beans

Cannellini beans

black beans

Kidney beans

Black eyed peas

Pinto beans

lentils

Soy beans

navy beans

great northern beans

Nuts + seeds - unsalted
Walnuts   Cashews

almonds   Brazil nuts

peanuts   Hazelnuts

pistachios   Pecans

pumpkin seeds

Chia seeds

Dairy
Cottage cheese

Ricotta cheese

Mozzarella cheese

unsweetened plain whole milk yogurt

unsweetened greek yogurt

Fruits
apples   avacado

blackberries blueberri-

Butternut squash

Cantaloupe Pears

Cucumber Tomato

mandarins

Raspberries

Strawberries

Vegetables

Spinach
Radishes
Brussels sprouts
Broccoli
Kale
Carrots
Bell Peppers
Cauliflower
mushrooms
asparagus
Edemame
Swiss Chard
Broccoli Rabe
Zucchini

Bonus foods

green olives
Cocoa nibs
Kale chips
guacamole
Cheese chips
unsweetened coconut
flakes
70% dark chocolate
pickles
Hummus
peanut butter
flaxseed crackers
bone broth

Lunch & Dinner bowls

✳ Pick one in each category

Beans

Chickpeas
Lima beans
Cannellini beans
Black beans
Kidney beans
Pinto beans
Lentils
Soybeans
Navy beans
great northern beans

Proteins

Eggs Tuna
Shrimp Chicken thighs
Salmon Tofu
Edamame
lentils
quinoa turkey
ground chicken

greens

Spinach
brussels sprouts
Broccoli
Kale
asparagus
Edamame
Swiss chard
Broccoli Rabe
Collard greens
Cabbage
arugula
bock choy
lettuce varieties
green beans

Made in the USA
Monee, IL
02 July 2020

1/2 C. beans
1 full cup greens
1 palm sized protein